GREEN UP YOUR MEDICINE

Easy Natural & Herbal Remedies & Recipes for Good Health

Green Up Your Life – Vol 4

By Pilar Bueno & Lucy Bond

**This edition published by
VIDDA Publishing Ltd in 2015. www.viddapublishing.com
Copyright © VIDDA Publishing Ltd 2015**

While the author has made all reasonable efforts to ensure that the information contained in this book is accurate and up to date at the time of publication, anyone reading this book should note the following important points:-

Medical and pharmaceutical knowledge are constantly changing and the author and the publisher cannot and do not guarantee the accuracy or appropriateness of the contents of this book;

In any event, this book is not intended to be, and should not be relied upon, as a substitute for appropriate, tailored professional advice. Both the author and the publisher strongly recommend that a doctor or other healthcare professional is consulted before embarking on major dietary changes;

For the reasons set out above, and to the fullest extent permitted by law, the author and publisher: (i) cannot and do not accept any legal duty of care or responsibility in relation to the accuracy or appropriateness of the contents of this book, even where expressed as 'advice' or using other words to this effect; and (ii) disclaim any liability, loss, damage or risk that may be claimed or incurred as a consequence - directly or indirectly - of the use and/or application of any of the contents of this book.

Cover design by John Hodges.

VIDDA Publishing BOOK SHELF:
www.viddapublishing.com/books.html

Have you thought about self-publishing via Amazon Kindle? If so to make the process easier and more productive, I highly recommend this software to help you on your way.

KBookPromotion: bit.ly/KBookPromotion

Your FREE Gift

Thank you for purchasing this book. To show our appreciation we would like to offer you a copy of our FREE recipe book "BRING LIFE TO YOUR FOOD". To download, visit our website: **www.viddapublishing.com**.

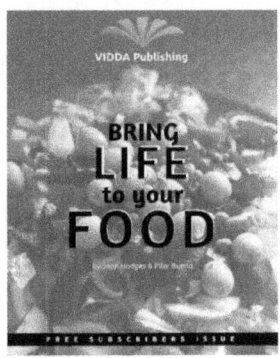

If you're interested in Health, Nutrition, Green and / or Cruelty-Free products please visit our Websites and online **VIDDA Health Stores** (US: bit.ly/VIDDAstore & UK: bit.ly/VIDDAstoreUK).

www.viddapublishing.com

www.sirtfood.com

www.themedicineonyourplate.com

www.greenupyourlife.org

www.ecologizatuvida.com

Table of Contents

Your FREE Gift..3

About this Book 6

Section 1: Why and How to Green Up Your Medicines -
Introduction 7
   Do We Need Proof? 8
   The Placebo Effect...10

Prevention Before Cure 12

Detoxing Your Body 14

Get Healthy...16
   Eat Well 16
   Exercise Regularly...19
   De-stress...19
   Get Good Habits 20

Green Up Your Medicine to Green Up the Planet...............22

Section 2: Practical Green Treatments...........................24
   Headaches and Migraines 25
   Colds and Flu 27
      Stuffy Nose 29
      Sore Throat 30
      Cough 30
      General Cold Symptoms.............................31
   Stomach Troubles 32
      Heartburn and Acid Reflux.........................32
      Constipation..34
   Girly Stuff...37
      Irregular periods 38
      Bloating 38
      Period cramp relief 38
      Thrush relief...39

Bacterial vaginosis 39

Skin Treatments 39

Dry skin conditions...40

Itchy dry skin 40

Spots and acne..41

Acne 41

Wet eczema...41

Blocked pores and greasy skin 41

First Aid 42

Bee Stings...42

Wasp stings 42

Sunburn...42

Small cuts 43

Toothache..43

Earache...44

Mouth ulcers 44

Conclusion 46

Before you go 48

Other Books by VIDDA Publishing 49

Connect with Pilar Bueno 52

About this Book

Are you fed up with minor little upsets in your body? Do you want to find ways of dealing with them that deals with the problem without leaving you with a dozen other problems instead? Do you want to do that in a way that's as natural as possible, without the use of potentially toxic chemicals and methods that are so often used in conventional medications and practices?

This book will introduce you to solutions that can help you to heal yourself with nature. In Section 1 we'll explain the reasons why greening up your medicines and your life is so important and can be rewarding. It shows you how you can get yourself as healthy as possible. Section 2 gives you the practical ways to deal with those minor problems and illnesses without "using a sledgehammer to crack a nut" – in other words how to use simple green and eco-conscious recipes and strategies to deal with everyday ailments.

The usual disclaimer here: we're not scientists and we don't know everything. The advice here is given in good faith, but part of taking control of your own health is becoming better informed. This book starts the ball rolling for you, but if you decide to follow any of these suggestions make sure you inform yourself as fully as possible before putting them into practice. If a problem is more than a minor one or doesn't go away, get professional help.

Section 1: Why and How to Green Up Your Medicines -

Introduction

The human body is a great thing, and we take it for granted. Until it stops working perfectly, that is. Once something goes wrong – such as we get pain or infection – we have a couple of different avenues we can go down.

- We can ignore it and let it get better on its own. Once upon a time that might have been the route people took. They let time be the healer, and often it worked. But we live in a society now where we look for instant gratification; we want something and we want it now. For one thing, we live such busy and hectic lives that we feel we can't manage to function under less than optimal health – ever heard someone say about a health problem "I don't have time for this." Ever said it yourself? I'm guilty as charged.

- We can get help from "professionals" for it. It's a scientific world we live in here in the West, and we've been brought up to believe that science can make us better, through an interaction of scientifically validated, commercially manufactured products and the intervention of a qualified professional who is trained and qualified to help. In other words, we "externalise" our health, and put it in the hands of someone else. For decades that's how we've treated health, but now evidence has proved again and again that the professionals don't always know best. Whether it's a lack of trust in the professionals brought about by media coverage and personal knowledge of mistakes and malpractice or a cynicism that results from a new understanding of the manipulation and "overselling" by the

7

big drug and pharmaceutical companies, many of us have lost faith in "The System's" ability to help us. Doctors and health professionals used to be held in very high esteem in our parents and grandparents eras – that's much less true now.

- Which bring us to a point that some of us have reached: a rejection of conventional practice and, a willingness to take our health and medication into our own hands, or at least into the hands of those that are not part of The System. In medicine, like in many things in our lives, we've started to look back at the lives of those that came before us, and realised that our new, scientific ways are not necessarily the great improvement that we thought they were, and we're looking to some of those old traditional ways for help. That's where this book is going to help you.

Do We Need Proof?

One of the problems with natural and so-called alternative remedies is the lack of good quality research on them. We know that people have been using them for years, centuries even, and presumably if that's the case, they must work – otherwise the well-known definition of Insanity comes to mind: "Insanity is doing the same thing over and over again and expecting different results"! I don't believe that whole generations of people before us were stupid. It's not just in the past that these remedies were the ones that people used on a daily basis either. There are whole regions of the world where people rely on natural products and remedies to treat themselves. I have a couple of theories as to why there isn't more good quality research that proves the effectiveness of some of these treatments and remedies.

The biggest issue is definitely that, in general, natural health and medicine doesn't make big money. We like to think that a nation of healthy people is a good thing, and governments certainly appear to push for that. But there is BIG money to be made out of "unhealthy" people – the pharmaceutical industry is a huge one, one of the biggest in the world. According to the World Health Organisation, the global pharmaceutical industry is worth more than $300 billion a year. Imagine a world where each person maximised their health and used natural remedies to treat their own ailments. It sounds great, but what about all those massive companies that produce our medications – what would happen to them (and to their shareholders) if people consistently treated themselves with products they could grow in their own gardens, or make with cheap easily available products? It's not just pharmaceutical companies that make money out of health intervention either – especially if you live in a country where healthcare is provided by private organisations.

Research into natural remedies often focuses on one particular aspect of a product – scientists take a single "active ingredient" and do their research on that. That's the way scientific research works – change one thing but keep everything else the same. But what if it's the combination of all the ingredients in a natural remedy that give the positive effects?

Because these are natural products, it's difficult to get consistency. The way the product is grown, collected and prepared means that there are different levels of the active ingredients in each batch – in the same way that one apple you eat might taste entirely different from the next, even though they're the same variety. This means it's difficult to prove (or disprove) any benefits a product might have because there are too many variables. Although conventional science may reject many of these natural medicines for this reason, a surprising number of synthesised pharmaceuticals are based closely on the active ingredients from natural plants – it may be more than coincidence that the natural sources can't be patented, but the synthetic versions can be (clue: patents are worth a LOT of money)!

In the interests of balance, I have to say it – the treatments and remedies might not work! Yes, they've been around for a long time, and our grandparents might have sworn by them, but that doesn't mean without a doubt that they work. Maybe the scientific proof isn't there because there isn't any proof? I don't believe that, and probably neither do you if you are reading this, but it's what some people will say, so we can't ignore it. I believe that the other reasons I give here are much stronger.

Testing an active ingredient of a natural product or substance in a laboratory on an animal is NOT the same as testing it in real life on a real person. Even testing on real people in unnatural situations, such as under the controlled scientific conditions that modern research requires, is not the same as the real-life use of the remedy. Also, the human being is complicated, and the body doesn't work alone – the brain and the mind are involved in all aspects of our lives. Which leads nicely into the next section.

The Placebo Effect

It's a phrase you'll often hear linked with a discussion about natural remedies, and it's usually used in a dismissive or derogatory way – "It's only a placebo effect". The placebo effect means that the product doesn't seem to have any active therapeutic effect that causes relief from symptoms; instead, it's the patient's expectations that they will get better by using the product that makes them recover. This theory is used against many natural remedies, as a way to discount them as valid. I don't know about you, but if I have a headache and I take something – natural or otherwise - to get rid of it, and it works, I'm happy! I don't really care if it is my mind and my expectation that makes it work, as long as the headache goes away. Let's face it: the chances are that it was some product of my mind that gave me the headache in the first place – stress or anxiety, for instance. The interesting thing is, even scientists acknowledge that products they think work because of the placebo effect actually produce real and measurable changes in the blood and body of the person taking them. For instance, in response to a placebo pain reliever, those in pain will show, along with a reduction in their pain, an increase in endorphins that counteract pain. A fascinating study that explains the placebo effect more fully can be found here: http://bit.ly/1MT7sGI.

Prevention Before Cure

"Prevention is better than cure" is a phrase that really comes into its own when we apply it to our health. If you want to make your health regime more green and eco-friendly, the very best thing you can do is to keep yourself as healthy as possible in the first place, using natural methods.

Your health is determined by many things that you can control, and we're going to talk about them later in the book – your diet, exercise routine, sleep, stress levels, habits. One other thing that you can control is the amount and number of harmful chemicals, which have been linked with asthma and more life threating diseases such as cancer, that you take into your body on a daily basis through every aspect of your life; from the food and water you are putting IN your body contaminated with pesticides, vaccinations and growth hormones, to other toxic chemicals you put ON your body such as cosmetics and personal hygiene products, not to mention the chemicals we use to clean and deodorize our homes. Greening your health means doing away with some of the commercially available over the counter medications for common ailments such as colds, headaches, indigestion, etc. that introduce these chemicals into your body, but it also means doing away with these toxins in other areas of your life as previously mentioned. We'll show you the importance of doing that. In the later chapters, we're going to get practical and tell you how to deal with some of the common minor disorders that can make your life miserable, without resorting to pharmaceuticals.

If you're looking for some relief, right now, from a specific problem, feel free to skip straight to the later sections. But make sure you come back and read the rest too, there's lot's of (healthy) food for thought here that will help you to green up your health and your whole life!

Detoxing Your Body

Diets and eating plans that are designed to help you "detox" are all the rage just now, but that's not what we're going to talk about here. These diets are to rid your body of the by-products of digestion from your food, a job the body does pretty well naturally when in optimum health – that's the purpose of your liver and kidneys, and ultimately your urine and "poo"! But when your system is overloaded with toxins, which leads to ill health, a detox diet full of nutrients, soluble fibre and water will help reboot your immune system.

What we're going to talk about is something different: detoxing from the toxins that are introduced into your body through your daily living in the products you use and come into contact with throughout the day. We're talking about chemicals and substances in your cleaning products, plastics and materials you handle, beauty products and personal hygiene products you use. These are elements and compounds that your body CAN'T break down. They're man-made, or else "natural" in the sense that they come from nature (such as oil-based petrochemicals, or minerals that have been mined), but they are not substances that were ever intended to be present in the human body. Even if the human body was as adaptive as we like to think it is, and eventually learned to deal with these chemicals, it would take thousands of years of evolution to get to the state where we developed the mechanisms to do that. And most of these substances have only been around for the last 100 years at most.

I hope you're not too disappointed if I tell you I don't have any magic remedies to help you clear these substances out of your body right now. For many of them, time will do that – they'll break down (although they might take years to do that) or be expelled so that gradually your body will be detoxed. But that's only going to happen if you don't put MORE of them into your system, and that is one of the basic aims of green living – to stop that toxification (I'm not sure that's a real word, but it describes what's happening) in your body, and those of your family and loved ones.

Now this book is about your medicines, I know, but it's about your health too. These poisons (that's what a toxin is, a poison) don't just sit there in your body inertly, they impact on it and interfere with its functioning in lots of ways. They trigger reactions and confuse systems so your body no longer works in the way that it's meant to, which leads to health problems, so it's entirely appropriate to be talking about greening your whole life in the context of greening your medicines. At a basic level, better health means less medicating and treating ailments, and reducing the number of toxins you take in is going to give you better health.

A lot of the toxins I've been talking about are taken into your body accidentally – you absorb them through your skin when you're using products, or inhale them or accidentally ingest them. But medicines are different. You DELIBERATELY take them, and they are produced to bring about changes in your body. Unfortunately, though, some of those changes lead to other changes too, and that leads to side effects of the medication. So, you might take something else to stop the side effect, and so on. Are you starting to see the downward path here?

So detoxing the rest of your life is probably the number one way to detox from your medicines – because you'll need a whole lot less of them. Check out our other books on ways to do that on the VIDDA Publishing website.

Get Healthy

In the same way that detoxing is going to reduce your reliance on treatment and medication, getting your body into a healthy state is going to do that too. That doesn't mean you're never going to need any treatment. Everyone gets aches and pains, infections and diseases, even the healthiest person – but there's no point in making it more likely!

This isn't a diet or exercise book, so we're not going to go into depth here. There's plenty of information available if you want to go deeper (I recommend checking out the book series The Medicine on your Plate currently available on Amazon), but for now here are just some of the basics, to jog your memory a little.

Eat Well

This isn't easy for two reasons:

It's just not easy! There are so many foods available to tempt us, even though we know they're not good for us. It's true that many of our favourites are unhealthy. In the same way that we talked about the way that big business makes money out of supplying us with synthetic drugs, there is also a massive food industry that makes money from producing and selling processed and packaged food.

There's a lot of conflicting advice. Every week brings out a new diet; one week it's more carb. less fat, the next week that's turned on its head. Some of these, like SIRT FOOD, have strong scientific-backed research (and incidentally meet most of the criteria for "sensible" eating that we talk about below). But others are more questionable. What this means though is that because we're not sure what is the best, we tend to do nothing and stick with our old ways, like rabbits frozen in headlights!

Not knowing is only part of the problem, we are also "victims" of society's current Fast Food culture. The majority of the ready-made processed "junk" foods we consume can be quite addictive. Our bodies quickly get used to the artificial sweeteners and "naughty" ingredients in them and soon crave for more. Have you ever wondered why often you feel hungry relatively soon after eating what looked like a satisfying meal? Your body is simply craving for nutrients that you did not get in the correct quantity from your indulgent meal. Our heavily processed foods are depleted of nutrients, so no wonder when you eat "rubbish" you feel like "rubbish".

Although diets differ in lots of ways, the easiest thing to do is to stick with the basics they all have in common. That way you can't go wrong, even if by next week there's a new fad in the news. So that means:

- Plenty of vegetables, especially green leafy ones. Go for lots of other different colours too, as each colour is linked with specific vitamins and minerals.

- A fair amount of fruit. Fruit has sugars in it I know, but these are natural sugars, not ones that have been refined and added. Have it in as natural a state as possible – if you can just munch on it without doing a thing to it except for washing it, so much the better.

- Nuts and seeds. Just about every diet includes these, so they can't be bad! They are full of vitamins, minerals, and good fats – why would you not want to eat them?

- Unprocessed meat and fish. Buy as good a quality (organic and from sustainable sources) as you can afford, and stick to meat in its natural state rather than something that has lots of (potentially unhealthy) additives. My advice is to go with variety too, that way if you've made a terrible mistake and 6 months down the line the information changes and you shouldn't be eating beef, or chicken, or salmon or whatever, at least you haven't been eating it every day! If you're vegetarian you'll have other sources of protein (such as dairy, beans, seeds, and nuts) but, not many people know, dark green leafy vegetables are huge sources of protein. Think of large strong mammals in the animal kingdom like the gorilla or cow: where do you think they get their protein from to grow to that size? Once again, go for variety but if for whatever reason you don't get that, introduce dietary supplements such as spirulina and wheatgrass (juice or powder).

- If you're eating grains, make sure they're whole grains – any other sort has had so much stripped from it that you might as well eat paper!

- Steer clear of artificial anything!

- Read labels, and learn what they mean.

- Experiment. We said at the beginning of this section that our favourite foods are often the unhealthy ones. Try to change this by trying new foods until you find healthy ones that become something you would choose as a treat over those bad foods.

Exercise Regularly

You knew this would be here, didn't you? Exercise regularly doesn't mean exercise for hours, though. The new way of thinking is that short sharp bursts of exercise are more effective than a long slog, which is just fine by me!

It doesn't have to be formal exercise either. If you want to go to the gym or out for a run, that's fine. But housework, gardening, playing a physical game, or going for a walk are all getting you moving, stretching and exercising your heart and lungs too. This is a change to your way of life if you don't normally exercise much, so you have to ENJOY it to keep it up week in and week out for as long as you can.

De-stress

This is another one you probably saw coming. More and more illnesses are being linked with stress, apart from the ones we've known about for years, like heart attacks and strokes. Lesser conditions like eczema, asthma, and IBS (irritable bowel syndrome), have all been linked to a stressful life, and it's even been implicated in serious conditions like cancer – this scientific paper (http://bit.ly/1M7H1yl) explains how (also see the Amazon book *The Medicine on your Plate - Crushing Cancer*). I know this is easier said than done. A lot of sources of stress can probably be easily removed from your life with a bit of common sense, a new perspective or change of attitude towards it. However, other serious sources of stress might not be so easily eradicated from your life, so if you can't remove them completely from your life or escape from them, learn better ways to cope, embrace or live with it. So how can you de-stress?

- Make it a priority. Saying you don't have time to do it is like saying that your health (and so you) aren't important enough to be at the top of your "to-do" list.

- Make it achievable. There's no point saying you're going to start meditating every day, or go to yoga, or whatever you choose, if you know you won't have enough time to block out for it on a regular basis. Much better to choose something you know you can fit in regularly, and stick with – just like the exercise advice above.

- Cheat! Learn ways of relaxing and letting go that you can do at any time, in the middle of whatever else you're doing. A little bit of long slow breathing can be done at a desk, sitting at traffic lights, standing in the checkout queue or anywhere else you find yourself with a couple of minutes.

- Find what fits. The best way to distress is to do what YOU love to do, not what someone else tells you that you should. If it's gardening or playing the guitar or reading a book or taking a walk, as long as it relaxes you, gets you "in the moment" and gives you a bit of perspective on life, it's a winner.

Get Good Habits

As well as exercise, diet, and stress, our other daily habits influence us too. The two biggies are smoking and drinking. Whatever scientific research might disagree on, the one thing it absolutely agrees on is that smoking is a killer. You're taking those horrible toxins we're talking about into your body numerous times every day, and they're doing damage of course. But also, if you carry on smoking you'll find it much harder to justify making any of the other changes to green up and detox your life – they are all going to seem a bit pointless if you continue to poison yourself with cigarettes.

The same goes for alcohol too. The effects are less obvious, but they are still there. Moderation is the key – we're not asking you to give it up, just to keep an eye on your intake. If you ever ask yourself, or anyone else, the question "Am I drinking too much?" that probably means the answer is "Yes".

Green Up Your Medicine to Green Up the Planet

No discussion about greening your life can ignore the effects that conventional products have on the planet too. It's true that detoxify your medicines and the rest of your lifestyle can be great for you, but it also reduces the environmental impact of your healthcare and daily living.

Pharmaceuticals get into our ecosystems, particularly marine and water-based systems in a couple of ways, according to scientists. One study (http://bit.ly/1jAiohu) shows that increasing use of antihistamines and other medications means that water courses are becoming contaminated, and this can disrupt the delicate balance of the ecosystems. Our sewage systems don't cope well with the influx of synthesised products that increasing use of pharmaceuticals brings, with the result that they escape into rivers and sea along with the "clean" water from sewage treatment. These drugs get into the water in the first place either during the manufacturing process or possibly due to simple excretion in the waste of users. Another source of contamination is people simply flushing unused drugs down the toilet! As well as affecting the ecosystem, these substances can also be recirculated back to us in our foods (especially if we're eating fish and shellfish). An issue of particular concern is the presence of antibiotics in wastewater. Several studies have shown this can lead to the development of antibiotic-resistant bacteria, which impacts greatly on the environment and gives concern that these can be passed back into drinking water. This has the risk of exposing us directly to these bacteria which may cause illness, and expose us to the possibility of other bacteria in our system mutating and becoming antibiotic resistant themselves. You'll find extra reading here (http://bit.ly/1FaO5GW) and here (www.purewatergazette.net/antibiotics.htm) if it's something you want to know more about.

One of the benefits of using the simple remedies we're discussing is the lack of packaging that they bring with them – a few simple substances are all that you need to create this natural pharmacy. That means that we do away with the need for extensive packaging and the accompanying literature that comes with most conventional medications. Even if these are recycled rather than sent to landfill, there is an energy cost in that recycling. Another energy cost of conventional medicines comes in the form of transportation. You'll benefit the environment by reducing the amount of both raw ingredients and the final packaged products that are being transported around the world – so you'll help reduce the use of valuable fossil fuels and prevent the associated air pollution. Another benefit, of course, is the money you'll save!

Section 2: Practical Green Treatments

Now we've looked at the reasons to green up your medicines and reduce reliance on synthetic medication, we can have a look at the practical ways to do it.

This is a good time for a word of caution. Nature isn't always benevolent – there are natural products that can harm us too. A simple example is the nettle. We can make a great diuretic tea from the leaves, and they're full of vitamins and minerals. But we know they can also give us a sore sting! How you prepare and use the products is important, and so is knowing what you're using. If you're going to forage for herbs and berries to use, make sure you know without a doubt what they are – and if in doubt, don't risk it. Nature is very good at mimicking in order to protect itself, and things that look very similar can have different effects – anyone who's seen the film "Into the Wild" must remember the scene where the main character forages for a wild plant and then realises that the one he's eaten is, in fact, a poisonous look-alike – and it kills him!

Some natural products still have side effects too. If you're using something and you develop a reaction or another problem, stop using it – that's common sense. When you're starting out on your path to using nature to heal, use the minimum doses and work your way up. We hope this little book will set you on the path to green medicine – we recommend that once you find a remedy that you're interested in using, you get more information on it. A bunch of herb leaves doesn't come in a packet with a giant sheet of paper telling you usages and side effects in the way that commercial pharmaceuticals do; you need to gain that knowledge for yourself – and you know what they say: "Knowledge is power".

Reading this and other books, and following that information, makes you more in control and gives you more power over your own life – that's a good feeling!

We know that the human body possesses an extraordinary ability to heal and auto repair itself. To learn to heal ourselves is to learn to trust and develop this healing capacity that we have that nobody taught us.

A major bonus of this natural path is a reduction in cost. You'll find something like lavender oil used again and again for treatment of many different types of condition. A bottle of good quality oil will cost about the same as one packet of branded pain relief tablets, but will be used dozens of times. So you're helping your budget too.

Headaches and Migraines

Everybody gets headaches at some time or other; some of us get them regularly. Many of us just put up with them, rather than take conventional medication, but it doesn't have to be an either/or choice – the third way is to use a natural remedy. If you get mild headaches fairly regularly, take a look to see if there's anything in your lifestyle that might be causing them, and deal with that too. One of the "usual suspects" is tension, especially if you're keeping your head and neck rigid – maybe working at a computer for a long time. Another cause is food – especially if your headaches are migraine-type ones: cheese, coffee, and chocolate are all common triggers.

As always, if your headaches are very regular or severe, take professional advice. But for the run-of-the-mill headaches that most of us get, here are some simple natural remedies.

Lavender oil. Sweet smelling and calming, lavender oil can be used for headaches in a couple of ways. Its one of the few essential oils you can use undiluted, so just rub a couple of drops onto your temples – the simple act of rubbing it in and massaging the temples will help. This is a good remedy if you're out and about. If you're at home, add a few drops of the oil to a bowl of steaming water, and inhale the steam (cover your head and the bowl with a towel to maximise the steam inhalation.

Peppermint oil for tension headaches. If your headache is a tension headache, try a few drops of peppermint oil in a steam inhalation. Peppermint oil has both anti-inflammatory and antispasmodic effects.

Ginger. This is especially effective for migraines as it is a powerful anti-inflammatory. It's thought that it may work on prostaglandins in the body, which can cause inflammation, including in the blood vessels supplying the head and brain. Pour hot water over three slices of ginger, about the thickness of a coin, and allow to infuse then drink the juice. You can crush the slices then strain if you prefer. Just chewing on a piece of ginger, or some crystallised ginger, will also help. As well as helping the headache, ginger is great for reducing nausea that often comes as part of a migraine.

Clove tea. Regular tea contains caffeine, which causes the blood vessels to constrict, which can sometimes help a headache. Cloves have the same effect, so mixing the two together gives double benefits. Just bruise 4-6 clove heads with a mortar and pestle or between the bowls of two spoons, and add to the tea.

Massage. Massaging the temples and the occipital area (the back of the neck) will help to reduce tension and increase blood flow.

Hot and cold compresses. It seems contradictory to use both heat and cold, but sometimes the headache can be caused by spasms in either the muscles or the blood vessel walls. The heat relaxes the tension in the muscles or vessels and acts as a kind of "reset", stopping the spasms. The cold then constricts the vessels. Apply the compresses either to the forehead, making sure you include the temples, or to the back of the neck just below the hairline.

Drink water. This one should really be at the top of the list because it's the easiest and also because dehydration is probably the main cause of headaches. I can't stress enough how important it is to keep hydrated to replace the fluids that we loose when we breathe, sweat or urinate, not to mention when we exercise (did you know our body is between 60% and 70% water?). Yes, we get some fluids from the foods we consume but most of it should come from drinking (aim to drink at least 2 litres of water a day). As a nice motivator, you should know that drinking enough water helps you burn fat and increase your energy levels and brain function. And guess what? It's FREE.

Colds and Flu

First, let's get it straight – colds and flu are caused by viruses. That means that antibiotics won't work on them. It also means you don't catch them by getting wet in the rain, or by washing your hair when you have your period, whatever your mum or granny might tell you. Treating a cold, or even flu relies on treating the symptoms, and maybe shortening its life. By helping to boost your immune system with high doses of vitamin C via fruits and vegetables you can kick start your own natural defences. A personal recipe that has been very effective for me and my family:

Take 2 large lemons 4 green apples and a large piece of fresh ginger (about 5cm) all with their skins on, and juice. Drink a large glass first thing in the morning and last thing at night. I have found this extremely effective within 24 hours of ingesting.

This book is about taking control of your medicines yourself, so we're not concentrating on supplements that you have to buy. But lots of people reach for Echinacea and vitamin C as soon as they have a cold. Echinacea is prepared from various parts of the plants of the same name. Research has found very slight benefits to taking it during a cold, primarily to shorten the length of the cold. If you need to know the science, you'll find it in this paper (http://bit.ly/1QRZ1eb), which also points out that research on Echinacea is problematic as each preparation varies widely in its concentration of active ingredients, depending on which part of the plant it's made from and the species of plant used. The study showed it had the same level of effect as a placebo in most cases – which doesn't necessarily mean it's not effective –check out what we said about the placebo effect in the first section!

Vitamin C is another common go-to with a cold, but again the scientific jury is out on its effectiveness. This research by the National Center For Biotechnology Information (http://1.usa.gov/1MT7D58) suggests that although results about it are conflicting, on balance and since there are few side effects, it is worth taking to shorten the length a cold lasts for. It seems to be better to take it regularly rather than just during a cold. So make sure to increase the intake of vitamin C in your diet. Traditionally we have turned to oranges as a great source of vitamin C but they don't have, by any means, as high concentrations of it as other fruits and vegetables, for instance, lemon, kiwi or most green vegetables. Get into a habit of squeezing some natural lemon juice into your water (for one thing, it makes the water taste more interesting). But if you really want a daily injection of vitamin C, put a whole lemon (including skin, as this is where the highest concentration of vitamin C is) in your green smoothie or juice.

Also, be aware that the symptoms of a cold are there for a reason. Your temperature goes up because you're fighting the infection; your nose runs because the mucous in there is "trapping" the germs. That means that if you can put up with them, you're better to leave these symptoms alone – they're part of your body's defence mechanism. If they're just too unpleasant to put up with, though, try some of these remedies.

Stuffy Nose

Nostril wash. Mix ¼ teaspoon each of salt and baking soda in about ½ pint of warm water. Hold one nostril closed by applying light finger pressure while squirting the salt mixture into the other nostril with a syringe or nasal aspiration kit. Allow the liquid to drain, bringing with it dry mucus and dead microbes and cells (yeuch). Repeat two to three times for each nostril.

Nose Rub. For a nose that's sore and red around the nostrils, add a couple of drops of menthol or eucalyptus to a teaspoon of coconut oil. Rub with a spoon or your finger to dissolve the coconut oil. Apply to the outside edge of the nostrils. The eucalyptus/menthol is mildly numbing, and will also help clear the nose.

Sore Throat

Tea tree gargle. This uses the antiseptic qualities of the tea tree oil. Put 5-8 drops of tea tree oil in a glass of water. Gargle as far back into the throat as you can. Spit out – don't swallow, as tea tree is toxic.

Honey and Apple cider vinegar gargle. The vinegar is astringent, and tightens the membranes, reducing a tickle, and the honey soothes and coats the throat. Honey also has some antiseptic properties.

Make a mixture of 3 tablespoons of ACV, 1 tablespoon of honey, and 1/4 cup of warm water. Gargle 3-4 times a day with the mixture. It is also safe to swallow.

Tea toddy. This is good if you're restless at night because of all the symptoms of your cold. Make a cup of herbal tea, or regular decaffeinated tea. Add a tablespoon of whisky and a teaspoon of honey. Allow to cool slightly then drink. The whisky will help you sleep, and the honey will soothe your throat.

Golden turmeric milk. This combination of golden spices is antiviral and anti-inflammatory. Gently heat a cup of your preferred milk. While heating, add ½ teaspoon of turmeric, a crushed cardamom pod and ¼ teaspoon each of freshly ground black pepper and cinnamon. Sweeten with a teaspoon of honey, and whisk in a teaspoon of coconut oil to help the absorption of the spices into your system. Strain to remove the cardamom pod and drink warm.

Cough

This soothing and delicious tasting cough syrup uses the following ingredients: Honey, Lemon, Ginger, Pepper &

Thyme. Combining antimicrobial, antibacterial, anti-inflammatory and decongesting properties, it will soothe irritated membranes, help you loosen congestion and expel mucous as well as opening the airways by relaxing the muscles of the trachea and bronchi.

Mix 8 tablespoons of Honey (ideally Manuka) with the juice of 1 lemon.

Add 1 teaspoon of ground thyme, ground black pepper and ground ginger (if you have the fresh ingredients even better, but if so I recommend that you put them through the coffee grinder). Mix it all until you get an even smooth texture.

Transfer the mixture into a container for storage. If sealed properly and stored in a cold dry place it will keep for weeks.

Take a teaspoon every four hours when signs of first symptoms appear.

General Cold Symptoms

We have established how important it is to drink water to keep hydrated and more so when you have a cold / flu. This family recipe will help you dealing with your cold symptoms by improving your breathing and help you get rid of unwanted phlegm in your lungs. If you can, use fresh herbs but if not, dry herbs will also work. Here are the 3 wonder herbs and their properties:

Oregano: Antibacterial, antifungal, antioxidant, anti-inflammatory and antimicrobial

Thyme: Expectorant , antiviral, bactericidal, fungicidal, antibiotic and antiseptic.

Rosemary: Antibacterial, anti-inflammatory, anti-microbial and antioxidant

Boil 2 litres of filtered water on a saucepan. Turn the heat right down and add 2 large teaspoons of oregano, 1 teaspoon of thyme and 1 teaspoon of rosemary. Stir in, cover and turn the heat off. Let it rest for 10 minutes. Using a sieve, pour yourself a large mug and add some honey. Try to consume 2 litres a day.

Stomach Troubles

Digestive disorders can be uncomfortable and inconvenient (in a running to the loo sort of way). Digestive problems can include anything from one end of the system (such as acid burning in the throat) to the other (including constipation or diarrhoea). Tummy troubles are often a lifestyle thing, and can be caused by a variety of factors, including diet and stress. Acid indigestion can often be the result of eating the wrong diet, including diets high in refined sugars. Too much coffee, wine, or spicy foods can cause symptoms in some people. If you think yours might be diet related, keep a food diary to see if there's a relationship between what you eat and your bouts of heartburn.

Heartburn and Acid Reflux

These don't seem like major problems, but anyone who's had heartburn and acid reflux knows just how uncomfortable they can make you. Known by the grand name of Gastroesophageal Reflux Disease (GERD), it sounds like what it is – a condition where the stomach contents and acid come back up the oesophagus, causing the inner layer to be "burnt" by the acid, which gives inflammation just like you'd get after any acid burn. Lots of people think that it's the result of too much acid being produced, but that isn't necessarily true. It's caused instead by a malfunction in the sphincter at the lower end of the oesophagus, which allows the acid to flow back up. If you have persistent heartburn and need to keep using remedies, natural or otherwise, get it checked out as it could be a symptom of a hiatus hernia or of the presence of *H.Pylori* bacteria, which is implicated in stomach ulcers and also in the formation of some stomach cancers – it is treatable (although you might have to bite the bullet and go with conventional antibiotics on this one – it's an imperfect world). Natural treatments for heartburn and reflux include:

Aloe vera juice. This is a preparation made from the sticky sap of the aloe vera plant, which has any number of uses for health. The juice is anti-inflammatory, and drinking half a cup before meals will cool and reduce any inflammation in the digestive tract, and help to stop any food that irritates you from causing an inflammatory response. One problem with the juice though is that it has a laxative effect, so if you don't want this (you might if constipation is a problem), try one of the powdered products that have the laxative compound removed.

Slippery Elm. This comes from the inner bark of the tree of the same name and is found in the USA and Canada, among other places. Its long history of use goes back to the Native American Indians and the early American settlers. It has quite a number of therapeutic uses (have a look here for some of them: http://www.drugs.com/npc/slippery-elm.html) but the one we're interested in here is as a demulcent – which means that it forms a protective layer over a mucous membrane. That means that the gut is protected from acid and irritants passing through it. Note: it has been linked with miscarriage, and shouldn't be taken if you're pregnant. It comes in powdered form to add to water (or a water/milk mix), and can be taken either as a drink or in a thicker preparation as a thin porridge.

Whichever way you take it, do it immediately after preparation or it will become thicker and more of a paste if left to sit.

Chewing Spearmint or Peppermint Leaves. If you remember basic Biology from school, you know that the stomach contents are broken down by acid, to give an acidic solution. But saliva produced in the mouth is alkali, so producing saliva counteracts the acidity and reduces heartburn. Chewing makes you produce more saliva!

Constipation

Anyone who thinks constipation is funny has never had it – and that means no one! It makes you feel bloated, gives you stomach cramps, and since your poo (I know it's called faeces in the grown-up world, but I'm going to stick with poo, I think we'll all be more comfortable with that) carries lots of toxins and waste from your body, it "poisons" your system. This can make you feel sick and tired and give you spots, among other things. Laxatives are a huge market for pharmaceutical companies, but many of the products you can buy are based on natural products, so it makes sense to try the real thing, rather than something that has numerous chemicals and additives and is often stronger than it needs to be.

There are three main causes for minor constipation (assuming no underlying medical problem – as always, if it persists, get it checked out):

Your poo is too hard as it doesn't have enough water in it.

You're not making enough poo for it to stimulate your reflexes to expel it.

Your lower intestine and bowel isn't doing the work it needs to allow you to "go".

Different treatments are aimed at one of these three causes.

Water. Always start with the easiest and least intrusive treatment. As the waste from your digestive system travels along the gut, your system draws water out of it – otherwise, you'd have constant diarrhoea: very unpleasant. But if you don't have enough water in your system to supply all the cells and keep them plump and lush, more water will be drawn out of your poo, leaving it hard. This means that a) it moves more slowly through your system and b) it's really (I mean really) unpleasant to pass, so you fight nature and hold on tight. And as it sits there in your bowel MORE water is drawn out of it, making it even harder. So, long story short, make sure you're well hydrated, and that might be enough to solve the problem.

Another way to increase the water in your poo and make it softer is to draw the water out of the tissues through osmosis.

Magnesium. This works osmotically to draw the water through into the gut and so soften the poo. Foods that are high in magnesium include dark green leafy vegetables, seaweed, avocados, and nuts. If you increase your magnesium intake, make sure you increase your fluid intake too!

Increase fibre from food. This easy treatment is aimed at adding bulk so that your poo passes through your system more easily and also stimulates the gut to do what it has to do. Adding bulk naturally means adding fibre, the non-soluble sort. Dietary fibre should be tried first: beans, pulses such as lentils, whole grains, including oats (make sure they're unrefined though, instant oats have had nearly every bit of fibre stripped out of them), leafy vegetables, fruit – all things that are good for you anyway, and will give you lots of benefits for your health. And don't forget those prunes we all know about – and dried fruits including apricots and figs.

Flax Seed. Adding a couple of tablespoons of flaxseed to your daily diet increases the fibre levels (and gives you a good dose of omeaga-3 oils, which don't help your constipation but are great for you anyway). Sprinkle them over your cereal and salads.

Smoothies. You can increase your fibre with fruit and vegetable smoothies. By taking a smoothie rather than fruit or veg juice, you get all the fibre that the fruit has. Add your flax seed into your smoothie to increase your fibre even more.

There are some things that will naturally stimulate your gut if it's acting slowly, and cause it to contract and push your poo along.

Coffee. A strong cup of coffee will often do it – the caffeine stimulates the intestine. Don't overdo it though as caffeine has a diuretic effect, so can leave you dehydrated, which will counteract the positive effects

Another group of substances that have the same effect are those that contain anthraquinones (as they have an irritant or laxative effect on the large intestine), which include rhubarb root, buckthorn, senna and aloe vera (this information comes from a VERY detailed study on the effects of laxatives, which you can find here: www.itmonline.org/arts/laxatives.htm).

Rhubarb root tea. Combine a teaspoon of ground rhubarb root with about 8oz of hot water. Add organic honey preferably or black strap molasses as it's quite bitter. Rhubarb root is one of the best sources of anthraquinones.

Aloe vera juice. Drinking aloe vera juice helps but note that other aloe vera products for constipation that you can buy from herbalists come from the leaf of the plant and can cause cramping so should ONLY be used for severe constipation as a last resort.

Standing and moving. The simple act of moving around encourages the muscle contractions that the gut needs, partly because it gives it the space to do it, which sitting hunched up in a chair doesn't.

Girly Stuff

If you're a man reading this, feel free to skip this chapter – we won't judge you.

We, women, have to cope with a few problems the men don't, like periods and menopause (and bad hair days; men don't seem to have those either). Periods can bring pain, and heavy bleeding, and bloating and just a feeling of "bleuch" – I know that's not a real word. Menopause has its own joys – if you're there, you'll know what they are. Unlike many of the emergency measures you'll find in this book, these need ongoing care and attention, either every month or for a long length of time. That means that it's even more important to be treating these naturally, without toxic chemicals if you can.

Basil tea. Crush up a handful of basil leaves and add to a cup of boiling water. Add honey too if you prefer it sweeter. Cover and leave it to cool. Sip from it over an hour or two to relieve the cramps. Basil contains caffeic acid, similar to caffeine, and is a pain reliever.

Fennel tea. Add a teaspoon of fennel seeds to boiling water, allow to cool and then drink. Start this a couple of days before your period starts. Fennel has antispasmodic and anti-inflammatory qualities.

Flaxseed. Sprinkle two teaspoons of flaxseed on your cereal or salad, or add it to a smoothie. It helps to control the levels of progesterone and can help reduce the length of your period.

Papaya and banana smoothie (why not add your flaxseed to this too?). Papaya contains anti-inflammatories that reduce cramps, as well as being a great source of vitamins and minerals. Bananas contain magnesium, which helps control cramps, and gives a good slow release of energy, to stop spikes in your blood sugar that can make you feel even more tired than you already are.

Irregular periods

Eat foods that are high in phytoestrogens. These mimic the body's oestrogen and help to make your cycle more regular. These foods include organic soya, nuts and seeds and green vegetables.

Bloating

Bloating is caused by retained water, so eat foods that have a diuretic effect. These include pineapple, tomatoes, cabbage, leeks, celery, carrots, parsley and cranberries.

Period cramp relief

Add a few drops of all the following oils to a carrier oil such as coconut oil, and rub on your lower stomach (and on your lower back if you feel your cramps there too): peppermint, clove, eucalyptus, cinnamon. They create a natural "tiger balm" muscle rub, without the petroleum base, as they act as vasodilators - the area will start to feel warm as an effect of the oils increasing the blood flow, which helps the muscles to relax. Do a skin test patch on a small area before rubbing over a wider area.

Thrush relief

Thrush is an infection caused by the *Candida* organism. It's common to carry the organism, but at times an imbalance happens that means it can multiply quickly and give us thrush symptoms. To rebalance the bacteria in your system, natural LIVE yogurt, containing bacteria that restore the balance can be used – and yes, if you've heard about this and wondered, you DO put it "down there"! Easy ways to apply it are either using a simple syringe, or smearing a tampon liberally with the yogurt, inserting it, and then taking it out, leaving the yogurt behind.

Bacterial vaginosis

Similar to thrush, this is a vaginal infection caused by an increase in a particular bacteria, *Gardnerella Vaginalis,* and can cause discharge and soreness. Aloe vera gel (100% natural with no added preservatives or preferably taken directly from the plant) is both antibacterial and soothing. Use it both externally and internally to bring relief. We suggest you do a small test first before using copious quantities.

Skin Treatments

Our skin takes a lot of flak daily and sometimes suffers because of it. There are also many conditions that can affect it – some of them man-made, like contact dermatitis, and others of them due to factors like genetics or hormones such as eczema or acne. A greener lifestyle, using more natural products and fewer chemical and petroleum based ones is one of the best moves you can make to start to treat a skin condition that you or a family member has. That's not just natural health treatments like these, but also natural products around your home for washing and cleaning, and even natural beauty products. Switching to these types of products will often clear up skin conditions you thought you and your family were stuck with. That's especially important if you've been treating these conditions with conventional creams and lotions, or even tablets – which means you've been taking in even more toxins and chemicals that could be affecting your health (for more information, check out the other books in this series).

Skin conditions vary among people in how they show themselves, for instance, some people with eczema may have a "dry" type, whereas others have "wet" eczema, where the sores weep and go crusty. Like every other sort of treatment, you'll need to experiment with these natural treatments to see which ones work for you and which ones don't.

Dry skin conditions

Coconut oil is the go-to for every skin condition (except maybe acne); as well as being wonderfully moisturising, this is also mildly antiseptic and anti-inflammatory. Just rub it onto the area regularly to keep it softened.

Itchy dry skin

Oats are a bit of a miracle food, and they're also great for itchy skin conditions – not just by eating them, but by bathing in them. I'm not talking about a bath full of porridge here, don't panic. Instead, put a cup of oats into a muslin bag (or even into a sock if you can tie it to stop them escaping) and put it into a hot bath. When the bath has cooled enough for you to get in, the water should be milky and soft. It cools off any itching and leaves the skin feeling soft and silky. The starch in the oatmeal dissolves in the water and coats the skin to prevent moisture escaping, which reduces the dryness and the itching.

Spots and acne

We know that tea tree oil is antiseptic and astringent. To treat spots, you can dab on neat for optimum effect on the affected areas, but if you have sensitive skin, dilute the tea tree in a little carrier oil such as vitamin E oil (approximately 5 drops in 10 ml of carrier). If in doubt, carry out a skin patch test before use.

Acne

Green tea is good for us if we drink it, but you can also use it on the skin to treat acne. It reduces inflammation and oil production, and calms and soothes the skin too. Make a cup of strong green tea, allow to cool and then dip a thin cloth in and squeeze out the excess. Apply to the skin and leave in place for a couple of minutes.

Wet eczema

Although most skin conditions benefit from moisturising, wet eczema is one that gains from being dried out. A sea salt spray can do this. Add a teaspoon of pure sea salt to ½ pint of water in a spray bottle. You can also add a couple of drops of lavender oil too if you like. This will work if you're one of those who find that your eczema is improved by splashing in the sea.

Blocked pores and greasy skin

Acne can be caused by excess grease production combined with bacteria in the skin's pores. Apple cider vinegar treats both of these since it's astringent and antibacterial. Dilute 1 cup vinegar with 2 cups water and wipe over the skin once or twice a day. As a bonus, it contains antioxidants that can help to reduce skin cell damage too.

First Aid

Accidents and unfortunate events happen, more to some than to others! Having a few of these remedies to hand can stop a little drama from turning into a crisis, without having to resort to over-the-counter remedies. Because most of them use basic ingredients that you'll have to hand if you are following our advice, you won't have one of those moments where someone has a sting and you've got no sting cream and will burn cream do the same thing, or should you use the antiseptic cream instead?

Bee Stings

Bee venom is acidic, so you want something to neutralise that acidity. Add a teaspoon of bicarbonate of soda to half a cup of water, apply to a cloth and hold on the sting (bees can leave their sting in, so check first — if it's still there remove it with tweezers).

Wasp stings

These are alkaline, so you need an acid to neutralise them. Plain vinegar will do the trick just fine — just dab on the sting.

Hold an ice cube or ice pack onto the sting. It numbs the nerves that cause the pain.

Sunburn

Aloe vera is perfect for cooling and soothing sunburn, as long as the skin hasn't blister or broken. If you have a plant, use the jelly-like sap from the leaves, just smearing it onto the area. Otherwise, you can buy gels, but make sure they don't contain added chemicals.

Small cuts

The body deals with cuts in its own time, producing platelets and coagulants to stop the bleeding. If you don't want to wait, though, here are a few methods to quicken the process – I can't guarantee that they're all pain-free (especially the cayenne pepper!).

- Hold an ice cube over the cut (as long as you're sure there's nothing in the cut). The cold will numb the pain receptors, and the blood vessels will constrict to cut off bleeding.

- Sprinkling some cayenne pepper or some turmeric over a cut will quickly stop the bleeding – although it nips a bit too! Not recommended for children!

- Both Lavender and tea tree oils speed healing and kill germs. You can apply either one of them directly to cuts and scrapes - it usually causes no pain.

- The best remedy for cuts is raw honey (in particular, Manuka honey) used over 2000 years to prevent and heal infections due to its antibacterial properties. Simply apply raw honey on the cut and cover up.

Toothache

One of the worst pains there is; if it lasts see a dentist as there may be a tooth fracture or cavity that needs treating.

Cloves. To relieve the pain, and reduce any infection, grind a few cloves up and mix into a paste with water. Either apply directly to the offending area on a small piece of cotton wool or add to warm water and gargle with it.

Garlic. If you dare try it, garlic is great for toothache as it contains the enzyme allicin, which is antibacterial and anaesthetic. Just crush up a clove and apply directly to the tooth - this might be best for people who live alone, and be warned, it can burn, so only put over as small an area as possible!

Earache

Only treat an earache at home if you're sure there is no chance of there being a perforated eardrum!

Olive oil. Warm a teaspoon of olive oil, tilt your head and pour the oil directly into the ear. The heat will soothe, and the oil will lubricate and soften any ear wax that might be causing a problem.

Onion juice. Grate an onion then squeeze out the pulp and collect the juice. Dribble this into the ear. It has antiseptic properties and will help to kill any bacteria that are causing infection. Do this twice a day.

Mouth ulcers

These are often caused by biting the inside of your mouth, which then gets infected. Sometimes they just arise unexpectedly, with no apparent reason.

Salt water rinse. Add a tablespoon of salt to a cup of water, and stir to dissolve. "Sloosh" it around your mouth, where the salt will help to draw liquid out of the affected area and so reduce inflammation.

Ice cube. Put an ice cube into your mouth and hold it against the ulcer. The cold will numb the pain and help reduce inflammation.

Cayenne rub. Mix a teaspoon of cayenne pepper to a paste with a little water, then dab on the ulcer. It sounds gruesome, but cayenne contains a substance called capsaicin, which disrupts the pain process and helps to numb the pain.

Conclusion

Before you started reading this book, maybe you had vague ideas about wanting to green up your medicines and treatments. I hope by now you've seen how this can be important for any number of reasons. Maybe you see how it ties in with greening up your life more generally too, making yourself healthier so that you can reduce the amounts of any treatments you need, and detoxing your whole life to reduce the number of toxic chemicals you are exposed to that can have detrimental effects on your body.

We've shown you that it doesn't have to be difficult – there's not much you need in your medical armoury to make any number of treatments for common complaints. And you've seen too that there's no need for overkill – a simple mild treatment is all you need in many cases, not the potent drugs and their side effects that come from major pharmaceuticals.

Remember that by going green and reducing your reliance on major pharmaceutical companies, you're taking responsibility for a major area of your life – your health – back into your own hands. Taking an eco-friendly approach to your health isn't just an airy fairy thing to do, it's powerful. I hope we've shown you that.

This isn't just about personal choice, though. Reducing the numbers of manufactured synthesised products you use right across your life is good for the planet too. We've talked about the effects on the environment of packaging and transport of pharmaceuticals. We've also spoken about the concern of antibiotic resistance, which is becoming an increasingly urgent problem that we need to find a solution for. By greening up your medicines, you can be part of that solution.

Good luck, and stay healthy.

Before you go

Thank you for purchasing my book!

If you found this book interesting and enjoyed reading it, I would really appreciate a short **review on Amazon**. All of your feedback is valuable to me, as your comments and input will be taken on board to help me make this and future books even better.

I would love hearing what you have to say. Please leave me a helpful REVIEW on Amazon.

Other Books by VIDDA Publishing

GREEN UP YOUR LIFE Series (Available in Spanish)
Take control of your health and well-being by introducing Natural, Eco-Friendly habits into your daily routine.

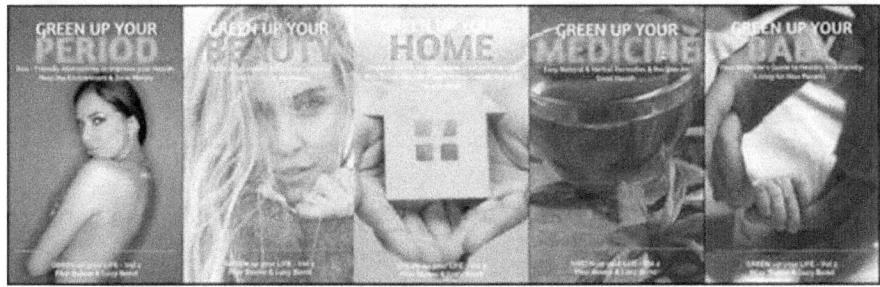

THE MEDICINE ON YOUR PLATE Series
Understanding Disease, Prevention & The Importance of Plant Based Nutrition and Diet

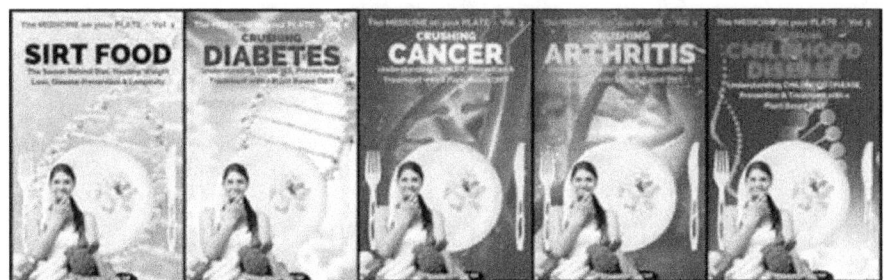

DOG TALES Series
Stories of Loyalty, Heroism & Devotion

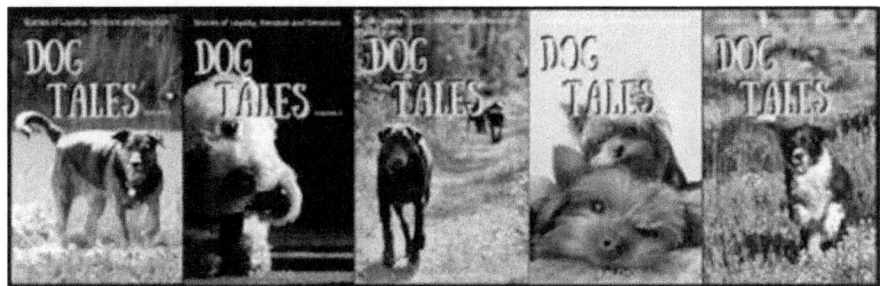

BUSINESS, INCOME & SOCIAL MEDIA Series
How to Promote, Market & Create Business with Social Media

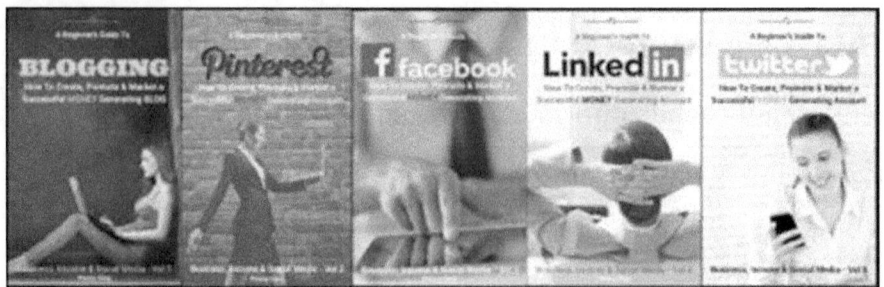

RESOLUTION TO BE HAPPY (Available in Spanish)
Make yourself smile every day and banish stress and anxiety forever

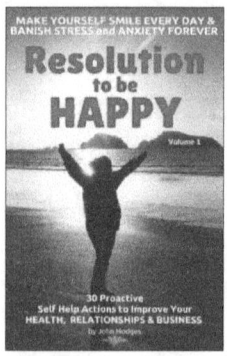

INTRODUCING GENETICALLY MODIFIED ORGANISMS - GMO
The History, Research and The TRUTH You're Not Being Told

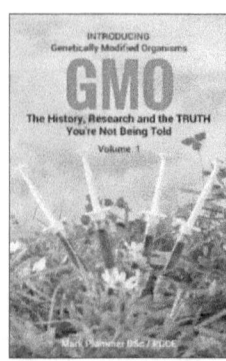

NATURAL WILD WINES

A Guide To Making Delicious Home Made Wine. Tips, Equipment, Recipes & Foraging Wild Fruits, Flowers & Herbs

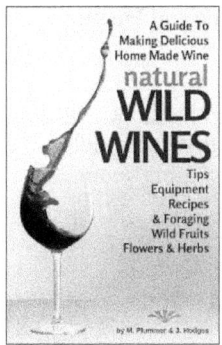

www.viddapublishing.com/books.html

Connect with Pilar Bueno

Thank you for taking the time to read my book. If it has helped you in any way or inspired you to introduce Greener and Healthier choices in your life, it makes me a very happy woman.

You can check out my publishing blog "Living like you mean it" (**viddapublishing.blogspot.co.uk**) for helpful tips, inspiration, and updates on new books and free promotions coming soon:

You can also follow me on:

Twitter: twitter.com/VIDDAPublishing

Pilar Bueno's Facebook: https://www.facebook.com/pilar.bueno.54

VIDDA Publishing's Facebook: www.facebook.com/viddapublishing

For your Healthy, Nutritious, Green and Cruelty-Free products, equipment and gadgets, visit our online **VIDDA Health Stores** (US: **bit.ly/VIDDAstore** & UK: **bit.ly/VIDDAstoreUK**).

Also, for our favourite supplier of nutrients, sprouting seeds and health products, visit **bit.ly/BuyWholeFoodsOnline**

If you have any questions at all, please feel free to contact me at: **viddapublishing.com/contact.html**

Wishing you a Green & Healthy Life.

 Pilar Bueno

www.viddapublishing.com

www.themedicineonyourplate.com

www.sirtfood.com

www.greenupyourlife.org

www.ecologizatuvida.com